Forward

Dear Reader,

Welcome to "Vibrant Transitions: Unleashing Your Vitality through Perimenopause and Menopause". This book has been meticulously crafted to empower you through the transformative journey of menopause, offering a holistic approach to reclaiming your vitality and embracing this new chapter in life.

Menopause is a natural and inevitable phase that every woman experiences, yet it often comes with its fair share of challenges and uncertainties. From fluctuating hormone levels and physical discomfort to emotional changes and lifestyle adjustments, it can be a turbulent time for many. However, it is essential to remember that menopause also signifies a new beginning, brimming with opportunity for growth and self-discovery.

In this comprehensive guide, we aim to provide you with the knowledge, tools, and guidance to navigate menopause with confidence, grace, and renewed energy. Drawing from the latest research, expert insights, and real-life experiences, we present a multidimensional approach that focuses on three key pillars: fitness, nutrition, and hormone balance.

Within these pages, you'll find practical advice on incorporating exercise routines that address menopause-related challenges such as bone density loss, weight management, and cardiovascular health. We delve into the benefits of various forms of physical activity, including yoga, strength training, and cardio exercises, tailored specifically to meet the needs of menopausal women.

A well-balanced diet is paramount during menopause, and our nutritional recommendations emphasize foods that support hormonal balance, improve mood, enhance sleep quality, and promote bone health. From superfoods and essential nutrients to meal planning and delicious recipes, we strive to simplify the journey toward optimal nutrition.

Understanding the intricacies of hormone balance is critical during this stage, and we demystify the complex interplay between hormones and menopause symptoms. We explore both conventional and alternative approaches, shedding light on hormone replacement therapy, natural remedies, and mind-body practices that can alleviate many of the discomforts associated with menopause.

Beyond the physical aspect, we delve into the emotional and psychological impact of menopause, acknowledging the profound changes and offering guidance on managing stress, enhancing self-care practices, and nurturing healthy relationships. By addressing the holistic nature of menopause, we believe you can embrace this as a transformative time of self-growth and self-acceptance.

Your journey through menopause should not be a lonely one. We are here to support you every step of the way on your path to reclaiming your vitality. Let this book be your guide, empowering you to make informed decisions, embrace self-care, and unlock your full potential during this significant life transition.

With warmth and dedication,

Petra Vaculik

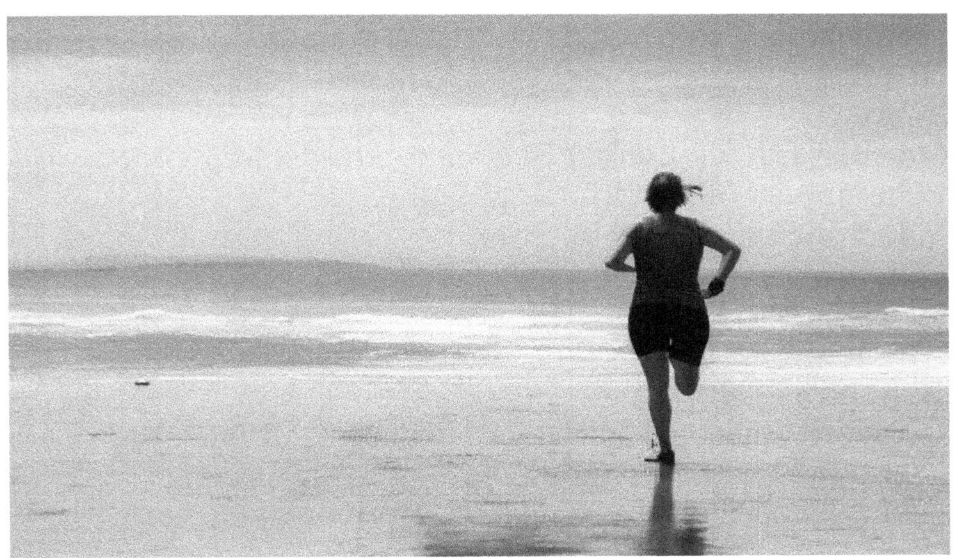

Table of Contents

Foreword

Chapter 1: Understanding Perimenopause and Menopause
- What is Menopause?
- Stages of Menopause
- Common Symptoms and Changes

Chapter 2: Hormone Balance and Perimenopause and Menopause
- The Importance of Hormone Balance
- Female Hormones and their Role in Menopause
- Hormone Replacement Therapy: Benefits and Considerations

Chapter 3: Fitness and Exercise for Perimenopause and Menopause
- The Role of Fitness in Menopause
- Types of Exercise: Strength Training, Cardio, and Yoga

- Acupuncture, Traditional Chinese Medicine, and Ayurveda
- Exploring Integrative Therapies

Chapter 10: Embracing Your Perimenopause and Menopause Journey
- Embracing Menopause as a Time of Personal Growth
- Resources and Support for Your Menopause Journey

Conclusion

Chapter 1: Understanding Perimenopause and Menopause

Menopause is a natural biological process that marks the end of a woman's reproductive years. It is a significant transition that every woman goes through typically in her late 40s or early 50s, although the exact timing can vary. Menopause occurs when the ovaries stop releasing eggs and the production of reproductive hormones such as estrogen and progesterone decreases significantly.

1.1 What is Menopause?

Menopause is often defined as the absence of menstrual periods for 12 consecutive months. However, the journey toward menopause starts years earlier with a phase called perimenopause. During perimenopause, which can last for several years, hormone levels fluctuate, and menstrual cycles may become irregular. Common symptoms experienced during perimenopause include hot flashes, night sweats, mood swings, and changes in libido.

1.2 Stages of Menopause

There are three stages of menopause: perimenopause, menopause, and postmenopause.

- Perimenopause: As mentioned earlier, perimenopause is the transitional phase leading up to menopause. It is characterized by hormone fluctuations and irregular menstrual cycles.
- Menopause: Menopause is officially reached after 12 consecutive months without a menstrual period. At this stage, the ovaries have stopped releasing eggs, and hormone levels have significantly decreased. Menopausal symptoms, such as hot flashes, vaginal dryness, and mood changes, may be more pronounced during this time.
- Postmenopause: Postmenopause begins after menopause and lasts for the remainder of a woman's life. During this phase, menopausal symptoms typically lessen, but the risk of certain health conditions, like osteoporosis and heart disease, may increase. Hormone levels stabilize at lower levels, and adjustments to lifestyle and healthcare may be necessary.

1.3 Common Symptoms and Changes

Menopause brings about various physical, emotional, and cognitive changes. While the experience can be different for each woman, some common symptoms and changes often associated with menopause include:

- Hot flashes and night sweats: Sudden feelings of intense heat, often accompanied by sweating and flushed skin.
- Changes in menstrual patterns: Irregular periods, lighter or heavier flow, or missed periods during perimenopause leading to the absence of periods in menopause.

- Vaginal dryness: Reduced lubrication and elasticity of vaginal tissues, leading to discomfort during sexual activity.
- Sleep disturbances: Insomnia, night sweats, and disrupted sleep patterns.
- Mood changes: Mood swings, irritability, anxiety, or depression.
- Changes in libido: Decreased interest in sex or changes in sexual desire.
- Changes in cognition: Some women may experience memory lapses or difficulty with concentration and cognitive function.

It's important to note that while these symptoms are common, not all women will experience them, or the severity and duration may vary. Understanding these symptoms and changes can help women navigate this transformational phase of their lives with greater awareness and readiness.

By familiarizing yourself with the process of menopause and its associated challenges, you can take proactive steps toward managing symptoms, maintaining good health, and embracing this new chapter with confidence.

Chapter 2: Hormone Balance in Perimenopause and Menopause

Hormone balance during perimenopause and menopause is a topic of great importance for many women. During this stage, the body undergoes various hormonal changes that can lead to a range of symptoms. Here are some key points about hormone balance during perimenopause and menopause:

1. Hormonal Shifts: Perimenopause is the transitional phase leading up to menopause, during which hormone levels, especially estrogen and progesterone, fluctuate. These fluctuations can contribute to a variety of symptoms such as irregular periods, hot flashes, night sweats, mood swings, and fatigue.

2. Estrogen Dominance: While estrogen levels decline overall during menopause, they can become relatively higher compared to progesterone levels, leading to a condition called estrogen dominance. Estrogen dominance can cause symptoms like breast tenderness, water retention, weight gain, and mood disturbances.

3. Progesterone Importance: Progesterone plays a crucial role in hormone balance during perimenopause and menopause. It not only helps regulate the menstrual cycle and support fertility but also helps counterbalance the effects of estrogen. Insufficient progesterone levels during this time can exacerbate symptoms related to hormone imbalance.

4. Lifestyle Changes: Making certain lifestyle changes can support hormone balance during perimenopause and menopause. These may include adopting a nutritious diet rich in fruits, vegetables, whole grains, and lean proteins. Regular physical exercise, stress management techniques such as meditation or yoga, and getting enough sleep are also beneficial.

5. Hormone Replacement Therapy (HRT): In some cases, hormone replacement therapy may be an option to alleviate symptoms of hormone imbalance. HRT involves supplementing the body with synthetic hormones, such as estrogen or progesterone, to rebalance hormone levels. It is important to consult with a healthcare professional to

understand the risks and benefits of HRT and to find a suitable approach.

6. Natural Remedies: Several natural remedies and supplements may assist in promoting hormone balance, such as black cohosh, red clover, maca root, and evening primrose oil. However, it's crucial to discuss these options with your healthcare provider before incorporating them into your routine.

Remember, hormone balance can vary between individuals, so it's essential to consult with a healthcare professional who can evaluate your specific needs and guide you towards appropriate treatments and lifestyle adjustments.

2.1 The Importance of Hormone Balance

Hormone balance plays a crucial role in maintaining optimal health and well-being. Hormones are chemical messengers in our bodies that regulate a wide range of bodily functions, including growth, metabolism, reproduction, mood, and sleep patterns. When these hormones are imbalanced, it can cause various health issues and disrupt the body's natural equilibrium.

Here are a few key points highlighting the importance of hormone balance:

1. Overall well-being: Hormones act as vital regulators in our bodies, contributing to our overall well-being. When hormones are in balance, we tend to enjoy better physical health, mental clarity, and emotional stability.

2. Reproductive health: Hormone balance is crucial for both men and women when it comes to reproductive

health. Imbalances can lead to fertility issues, irregular menstrual cycles, low libido, and even complications during pregnancy.

3. Energy and metabolism: Hormonal balance affects our energy levels and metabolism. When hormones like cortisol (which regulates stress) or insulin (which impacts blood sugar levels) are imbalanced, it can lead to fatigue, weight gain or loss, and poor metabolic function.

4. Mood and mental health: Hormones have a significant influence on our mood and overall mental health. Imbalances, such as low serotonin or dopamine levels, can contribute to mood swings, depression, anxiety, and other mental health disorders.

5. Bone health: Hormones like estrogen and testosterone play crucial roles in maintaining bone density. Imbalances, especially in women during menopause or in people with hormonal disorders, can increase the risk of osteoporosis and fractures.

6. Sleep patterns: Hormones like melatonin regulate our sleep-wake cycles. Imbalances can disrupt our ability to fall asleep or stay asleep, leading to insomnia or daytime drowsiness.

Maintaining hormone balance can be achieved through various approaches. Regular exercise, a balanced diet, stress management, and adequate sleep are essential lifestyle factors. Additionally, medical interventions and hormone replacement therapies may be required in certain cases, depending on the individual's specific needs.

It's important to consult with healthcare professionals, such as endocrinologists or gynecologists, who specialize in hormone health, if you suspect any imbalances. They can provide guidance, diagnose hormone-related conditions, and recommend appropriate treatments to restore balance.

Ultimately, prioritizing hormone balance is key to maintaining a healthy and vibrant life by ensuring the optimal functioning of our bodies' intricate systems.

2.2 Female Hormones and their Role in Perimenopause and Menopause

Female hormones play a vital role in perimenopause and menopause, as these stages mark significant changes in hormone production and balance. The key hormones involved are estrogen, progesterone, and follicle-stimulating hormone (FSH). Here's a breakdown of their role during perimenopause and menopause:

1. Estrogen: Estrogen is predominantly produced by the ovaries, and its levels fluctuate during perimenopause. As menopause approaches, the ovaries produce less estrogen. Estrogen is responsible for regulating the menstrual cycle, maintaining bone health, and supporting the health of the reproductive system. When estrogen levels decline, it can lead to various symptoms like hot flashes, night sweats, vaginal dryness, mood changes, and changes in bone density.

2. Progesterone: Progesterone works in tandem with estrogen to regulate the menstrual cycle and support fertility. During perimenopause, progesterone levels can fluctuate, resulting in irregular periods or skipped cycles. As menopause sets in, progesterone production decreases. Insufficient levels of progesterone can contribute to symptoms such as mood swings, irritability, water retention, and sleep disturbances.

3. Follicle-Stimulating Hormone (FSH): FSH is involved in the reproductive process. During perimenopause, FSH levels increase as the ovaries become less responsive to its signals. This increase can result in irregular menstrual cycles. High FSH levels are often used as an indicator of perimenopause or menopause transition.

4. Hormonal Interplay: Estrogen, progesterone, and FSH levels are interconnected during perimenopause and menopause. As estrogen levels decline, the normal balance between estrogen and progesterone can be disrupted, leading to symptoms of hormone imbalance. Changes in FSH levels also influence the fluctuation and irregularity of menstrual cycles.

It's important to note that the hormonal changes experienced during perimenopause and menopause are natural parts of the aging process. However, if the symptoms become severe or significantly impact daily life, it's advisable to seek medical advice. Healthcare professionals may recommend specific treatments or therapies, such as hormone replacement therapy (HRT) or other interventions, to manage symptoms and optimize hormone balance.

Remember, each woman's experience with perimenopause and menopause is unique, and it's essential to consult with a healthcare professional who can provide personalized guidance based on your specific needs and medical history.

2.3 Hormone Replacement Therapy: Benefits and Considerations

Hormone replacement therapy (HRT) is a treatment option that involves supplementing the body with synthetic hormones to alleviate symptoms of hormone imbalance, specifically during perimenopause and menopause. Here are some benefits and considerations to keep in mind:

Benefits of Hormone Replacement Therapy:
1. Alleviates Menopausal Symptoms: HRT can effectively relieve many symptoms associated with perimenopause and menopause, such as hot flashes, night sweats, vaginal dryness, mood swings, and sleep disturbances. It can provide relief for women experiencing severe or disruptive symptoms.

2. Improves Quality of Life: By reducing bothersome symptoms, HRT can significantly improve a woman's quality of life, allowing her to engage in daily activities without significant disruption. It can alleviate discomfort, increase energy levels, and enhance overall well-being.

3. Protects Against Osteoporosis: Estrogen helps maintain bone density, and the decline of estrogen during menopause puts women at a higher risk of osteoporosis. HRT can help preserve bone health and reduce the risk of fractures associated with osteoporosis.

4. Supports Heart Health: Estrogen has a protective effect on the cardiovascular system, and HRT may help reduce the risk of heart disease in certain women. However, this benefit may vary depending on individual health factors and the specific form of HRT used.

Considerations for Hormone Replacement Therapy:
1. Individualized Approach: HRT should be tailored to each woman's specific needs. It's crucial to consult with a healthcare professional who can evaluate your medical history, assess your symptoms, and recommend the most appropriate form and dosage of hormones for you.

2. Risks and Side Effects: Like any medication, HRT carries risks and potential side effects. These may include an increased risk of blood clots, stroke, breast cancer, and gallbladder disease. The risks can vary depending on a woman's age, health, and family medical history. It's important to discuss these potential risks with your healthcare provider.

3. Duration and Timing: The duration and timing of HRT can be individualized based on the severity of symptoms, overall health, and individual preferences. While short-term use of HRT is generally considered safe for symptom management, long-term use carries a higher risk of certain health conditions. It's advisable to regularly reassess the need for HRT with your healthcare provider.

4. Alternatives and Complementary Approaches: HRT is not the only option for managing symptoms of perimenopause and menopause. There are alternative treatments, lifestyle modifications, and natural remedies that may be effective for some women. It's important to discuss these options with your healthcare provider to determine the best approach for you.

When considering HRT, it's crucial to have an open and honest discussion with your healthcare provider. They can help evaluate the potential benefits and risks based on your unique circumstances, guide you through the decision-making process, and monitor your response to treatment.

Remember, HRT is a personal choice, and what works for one woman may not work for another. By working closely with your healthcare provider and considering all available options, you can make an informed decision about whether HRT is suitable for you.

Chapter 3: Fitness and Exercise

Perimenopause and menopause are stages in a woman's life that can bring hormonal changes and various physical and emotional symptoms. Regular fitness and exercise can play a crucial role in managing these symptoms and promoting overall well-being. Here are some key points to consider:

1. Strength training: As women age, they naturally start losing muscle mass. Engaging in regular strength training exercises can help counteract this process and maintain or even increase muscle mass. Resistance exercises, like weightlifting or using resistance bands, are particularly beneficial.

2. Weight-bearing exercises: These exercises help maintain bone density, which can decline during menopause. Incorporate activities such as walking, jogging, dancing, or stair climbing into your routine. Remember to use proper form and gradually increase intensity as your fitness level improves.

3. Cardiovascular exercises: Engaging in aerobic activities like cycling, swimming, or running can benefit cardiovascular health, manage weight, and enhance mood. Aim for at least 150 minutes of moderate-intensity aerobic exercise or 75 minutes of vigorous-intensity exercise per week.

4. Flexibility and balance exercises: Hormonal changes during menopause can impact joint and muscle health, leading to stiffness and a higher risk of falls. Include

activities like yoga, Pilates, or tai chi to improve flexibility, balance, and posture.

5. Mind-body exercises: Emotional well-being is essential during this transitional phase. Mind-body exercises such as yoga or meditation can help reduce stress levels, improve sleep quality, and promote relaxation.

6. Seek professional guidance: It's always a good idea to consult with a healthcare professional or a certified fitness trainer before starting a new exercise routine, especially if you have any underlying health conditions or concerns.

Remember, it's crucial to listen to your body and adjust the intensity and duration of your exercises accordingly. Stay consistent, find activities you enjoy, and set realistic goals to ensure long-term success. 3.1 The Role of Fitness in Menopause

3.1 The Role of Fitness in Perimenopause and Menopause

The role of fitness in perimenopause and menopause is crucial for maintaining overall health and managing the various physical and emotional changes that occur during this stage. Here's some key information about the role of fitness during perimenopause and menopause:

1. Hormone regulation: Regular exercise can help regulate hormone levels, including estrogen, which tend to decline during this stage. Exercise stimulates the production of endorphins, which can help improve mood and reduce common symptoms like hot flashes and mood swings.

2. Weight management: With age, it becomes more challenging to maintain a healthy weight due to hormonal changes and a slowing metabolism. Regular exercise,

improve sleep quality and alleviate symptoms such as insomnia.

3. Yoga:
Yoga is a particularly valuable form of exercise during menopause and perimenopause. It not only helps maintain flexibility, balance, and muscle tone but also supports stress reduction and relaxation. Yoga practice often incorporates deep breathing and mindfulness techniques, which can help manage anxiety, insomnia, and hot flashes associated with menopause. Certain yoga poses can also target specific symptoms like back pain, joint stiffness, and mood swings, making it a well-rounded exercise choice for menopausal women.

Overall, a combination of strength training, cardio exercises, and yoga can provide numerous benefits during menopause and perimenopause. However, it's essential to consult with a healthcare professional or a certified fitness trainer who can tailor an exercise program to your specific needs and abilities. Listening to your body, taking rest days, and gradually increasing exercise intensity is also important during this life stage.

3.3 Managing Weight, Bone Health, and Cardiovascular Health

Managing weight, bone health, and cardiovascular health are all important considerations during perimenopause and menopause. Let's go through each topic:

1. Managing Weight:
During perimenopause and menopause, hormonal changes can lead to weight gain, especially around the abdominal area. Here are some tips to help manage weight:

- Maintain a balanced diet: Focus on whole foods, including fruits, vegetables, lean proteins, whole grains, and healthy fats. Limit processed foods, sugary snacks, and drinks.
- Stay active: Engage in regular physical activity such as aerobic exercises, strength training, and flexibility exercises. This helps maintain muscle mass and boost metabolism.
- Be mindful of portion sizes: As metabolism slows down, paying attention to portion sizes can help prevent overeating.
- Get enough sleep: Adequate sleep plays a role in weight management. Aim for 7-8 hours of quality sleep per night.

2. Bone Health:
During menopause, estrogen levels decrease, which can lead to a gradual loss of bone density. To maintain and improve bone health:
- Consume calcium-rich foods: Include dairy products, leafy green vegetables, nuts, and calcium-fortified foods in your diet.
- Get enough vitamin D: Vitamin D is essential for calcium absorption. Spend time outdoors, expose your skin to sunlight, and consider taking supplements if your levels are low.
- Engage in weight-bearing exercises: Activities such as walking, jogging, dancing, and weightlifting can help strengthen bones.
- Avoid smoking and excess alcohol consumption, as they can contribute to bone loss.

3. Cardiovascular Health:
Menopause is associated with an increased risk of cardiovascular disease due to hormonal changes. Here's how to promote cardiovascular health:

- Adopt a heart-healthy diet: Focus on reducing saturated fats, trans fats, and cholesterol. Include fruits, vegetables, whole grains, lean proteins, and healthy fats.
- Engage in aerobic exercises: Aim for at least 150 minutes of moderate-intensity aerobic activity per week, such as brisk walking, swimming, or cycling.
- Manage stress: Chronic stress can impact heart health. Practice relaxation techniques like deep breathing, meditation, or yoga to reduce stress levels.
- Don't smoke: Smoking increases the risk of heart disease. Seek support or treatment options if you need help quitting.

Remember, these are general recommendations, and it's always a good idea to consult with your healthcare provider for personalized advice based on your specific health needs during perimenopause and menopause.

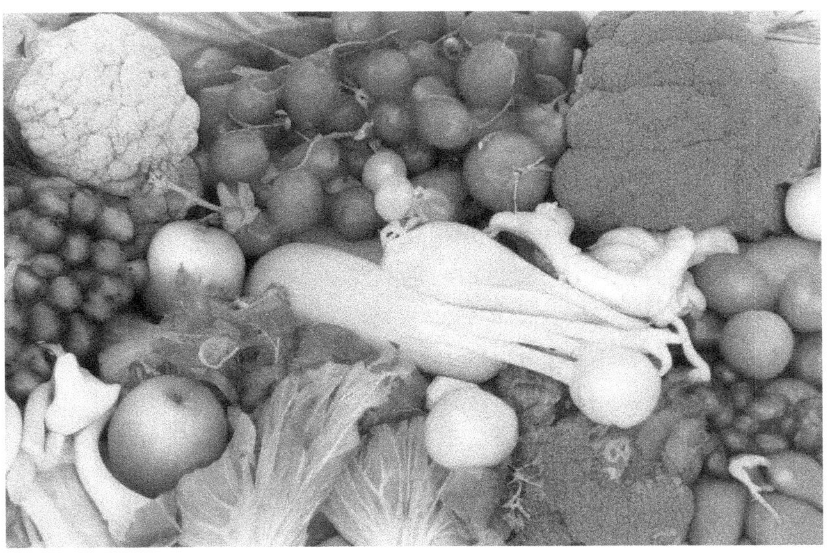

Chapter 4: Nutrition for Perimenopause and Menopause

Proper nutrition during perimenopause and menopause is crucial for managing symptoms and supporting overall health.

Remember, these are general guidelines, and it's always a good idea to consult with a healthcare professional or a registered dietitian for personalized advice tailored to your specific needs during menopause.

4.1 The Impact of Nutrition on Perimenopause and Menopause

Nutrition plays a crucial role in managing the symptoms of perimenopause and menopause and supporting overall health during this stage. Here are some key points about the impact of nutrition on perimenopause and menopause:

1. Balanced diet: Eating a balanced diet is essential during perimenopause and menopause. Focus on consuming a variety of nutrient-rich foods, including fruits, vegetables, whole grains, lean proteins, and healthy fats. Adequate protein intake is particularly important for maintaining muscle mass, which tends to decline during this stage.

2. Phytoestrogens: Phytoestrogens are plant compounds that have a weak estrogen-like effect in the body. They may help alleviate some menopausal symptoms by binding to estrogen receptors. Foods rich in phytoestrogens include soy products (tofu, tempeh, edamame), flaxseeds, sesame seeds, legumes, and whole grains.

3. Calcium and Vitamin D: Estrogen helps maintain bone density, and its decline during menopause increases the risk of osteoporosis. Adequate calcium and vitamin D intake is crucial for maintaining strong bones. Include calcium-rich foods such as dairy products, leafy greens,

and fortified plant-based milks. Additionally, getting regular sunlight exposure or taking vitamin D supplements can support optimal vitamin D levels.

4. Healthy fats: Consuming healthy fats is important for hormone production and overall well-being. Include foods rich in omega-3 fatty acids, such as fatty fish (salmon, sardines), flaxseeds, chia seeds, walnuts, and avocados. These fats provide anti-inflammatory benefits and support brain health.

5. Hydration: Staying hydrated is important for managing various symptoms, including hot flashes and vaginal dryness. Aim for at least eight glasses of water per day and limit your intake of caffeinated beverages, as they can exacerbate symptoms for some women.

6. Limit processed foods and sugar: Processed foods and added sugars can contribute to weight gain, inflammation, and mood swings. Minimize your intake of sugary drinks, packaged snacks, refined grains, and desserts. Instead, opt for whole, unprocessed foods to nourish your body and support hormonal balance.

7. Mindful eating: Practicing mindful eating can help you tune in to your body's hunger and fullness cues. Take time to savor your meals, eat slowly, and listen to your body's signals to avoid overeating. This approach can also help manage emotional eating, which can be triggered by hormonal fluctuations during perimenopause and menopause.

Remember, each woman's nutritional needs may vary, so it's advisable to consult with a registered dietitian or healthcare professional who can provide personalized recommendations based on your specific needs and health goals.

4.2 Macronutrients and Micronutrients for Optimal Health

During perimenopause and menopause, it's important to pay attention to your nutrition to support your hormonal changes and overall health. Here's some information on macronutrients and micronutrients that can be beneficial during this stage:

Macronutrients:
1. Protein: Incorporate sources like lean meats, poultry, fish, dairy products, eggs, legumes, and plant-based protein sources such as tofu or tempeh. Protein is crucial for maintaining muscle mass and supporting hormonal balance.
2. Healthy Fats: Include sources of monounsaturated and polyunsaturated fats like avocados, oily fish (salmon, sardines), nuts, seeds, and olive oil. These fats are beneficial for heart health and can help with hormone production.
3. Complex Carbohydrates: Opt for whole grains like brown rice, quinoa, oats, and whole-wheat bread to provide sustained energy and support gut health.

Micronutrients:
1. Calcium: Consuming adequate calcium-rich foods like dairy products, leafy greens (kale, spinach), legumes, and fortified plant-based milk can help support bone health, which becomes more important during menopause.
2. Vitamin D: Ensure you get enough sunlight exposure or consider supplements since vitamin D aids in calcium absorption and supports bone health.
3. Iron: Incorporate iron-rich foods like lean red meat, poultry, fish, legumes, and fortified cereals. Iron needs may

increase during menopause due to decreased estrogen levels.

4. Omega-3 fatty acids: Found in fatty fish, walnuts, chia seeds, and flaxseeds, omega-3 fatty acids help reduce inflammation and support heart health.

5. B vitamins: Include sources of B vitamins such as whole grains, lean meats, poultry, fish, legumes, and leafy greens. B vitamins play a role in energy production and neurotransmitter function.

Remember, it's always a good idea to consult with a healthcare professional or a registered dietitian/nutritionist who specializes in menopause for personalized advice based on your specific nutritional needs.

4.3 Superfoods for Hormone Balance and Overall Well-Being

While there is no specific definition of "superfoods," there are certain nutrient-dense foods that may support hormone balance and overall well-being during perimenopause and menopause. Here are some examples:

1. Flaxseeds: These tiny powerhouses are rich in lignans, which have estrogenic properties and may help balance hormone levels. They are also an excellent source of omega-3 fatty acids, fiber, and antioxidants. Add ground flaxseeds to smoothies, yogurt, cereal, or baked goods.

2. Soy: Foods like tofu, tempeh, soy milk, and edamame contain phytoestrogens called isoflavones, which have a weak estrogen-like effect in the body. These can potentially alleviate menopausal symptoms. Incorporate soy-based foods into your diet moderately.

3. Cruciferous vegetables: Vegetables such as broccoli, cauliflower, kale, Brussels sprouts, and cabbage contain compounds called indoles that support estrogen metabolism. They also provide a wealth of vitamins, minerals, and fiber that promote overall health.

4. Berries: Blueberries, strawberries, raspberries, and blackberries are rich in antioxidants and fiber. They support cellular health, reduce inflammation, and provide essential nutrients.

5. Avocado: This creamy fruit is an excellent source of healthy fats, including monounsaturated fats. These fats help with hormone production and absorption of fat-soluble vitamins. Avocado also provides essential nutrients like vitamin E and potassium.

6. Fatty fish: Cold-water fish like salmon, mackerel, sardines, and trout are high in omega-3 fatty acids, which have anti-inflammatory properties and support brain health. These healthy fats may also help alleviate menopausal symptoms.

7. Nuts and seeds: Almonds, walnuts, chia seeds, and pumpkin seeds are rich in healthy fats, fiber, and antioxidants. They can provide hormonal support and promote heart health.

Remember that a balanced and varied diet is key. Incorporating these superfoods as part of an overall nutritious eating pattern can support hormone balance and overall well-being during perimenopause and menopause. It's always a good idea to consult with a healthcare professional or a registered dietitian for personalized advice that takes into account any specific dietary needs or restrictions you may have.

Chapter 5: Meal Planning for Perimenopause and Menopause

Meal planning can be incredibly helpful during perimenopause and menopause to support overall health and manage any symptoms you may be experiencing. Here are some general guidelines and food recommendations that can assist in this journey.
5.1 Creating Balanced Meals for Hormonal Support

Proper nutrition is important during perimenopause and menopause to support hormonal health. Here are some tips for creating balanced meals:

1. Include a variety of whole foods: Make sure to incorporate a wide range of fruits, vegetables, whole grains, lean proteins, and healthy fats in your meals. These provide essential nutrients and help support hormonal balance.

2. Prioritize fiber-rich foods: Foods high in fiber, such as fruits, vegetables, legumes, and whole grains, can help manage hormonal fluctuations. They also promote regular bowel movements and help maintain a healthy weight.

3. Choose lean proteins: Including lean proteins like fish, chicken, turkey, tofu, and legumes in your meals can support hormone production. Protein is the building block for hormones, so it's essential to include an adequate amount in your diet.

4. Get good fats: Healthy fats like avocado, olive oil, nuts, and seeds are crucial for hormone production. They also provide satiety and support heart health. Avoid or limit saturated and trans fats found in processed and fried foods.

5. Include phytoestrogen-rich foods: Phytoestrogens, found in foods like soy products, flaxseeds, whole grains, and legumes, can help balance hormone levels naturally. However, it's essential to consult with a healthcare professional to determine the right amount for your specific needs.

6. Stay hydrated: Drinking an adequate amount of water each day is important for overall health and to support hormone balance. Aim for at least 8 cups (64 ounces) of water per day.

7. Limit processed foods and added sugars: Processed foods can contain harmful additives that disrupt hormonal balance. Similarly, excessive added sugar consumption can contribute to weight gain and hormonal imbalances. Aim to minimize your intake of these foods.

8. Manage portion sizes: Keep an eye on portion sizes to maintain a healthy weight. Overeating can lead to unwanted weight gain, which can worsen menopause symptoms. Be mindful of your portion sizes and listen to your body's hunger and fullness cues.

Remember, it's always a good idea to consult with a healthcare professional or a registered dietitian who specializes in women's health to create a personalized meal plan based on your specific needs and health goals.

5.2 Sample Meal Plans and Recipes

It's important to focus on nourishing your body and supporting hormonal balance during this stage of life. Here are a few ideas to get you started:

Sample Meal Plan for perimenopause/menopause:

Day 1:
- Breakfast: Spinach and mushroom omelet with whole grain toast
- Snack: Greek yogurt with berries and a sprinkle of nuts/seeds
- Lunch: Quinoa salad with mixed vegetables, grilled chicken, and a lemon-tahini dressing
- Snack: Sliced cucumbers with hummus
- Dinner: Baked salmon with steamed broccoli and a side of quinoa
- Dessert: A serving of dark chocolate with a handful of almonds

Day 2:
- Breakfast: Overnight oats with chia seeds, almond milk, and fresh fruits
- Snack: Celery sticks with almond butter
- Lunch: Mixed greens salad with grilled shrimp, avocado, cherry tomatoes, and a vinaigrette dressing
- Snack: Roasted chickpeas
- Dinner: Turkey meatballs with zucchini noodles and marinara sauce
- Dessert: Baked apples with cinnamon and a sprinkle of granola

Day 3:
- Breakfast: Vegetable and feta cheese frittata
- Snack: Roasted edamame beans
- Lunch: Lentil soup with a side of whole grain bread
- Snack: Carrot sticks with hummus
- Dinner: Grilled chicken breast with roasted sweet potatoes and asparagus
- Dessert: Mixed berry smoothie with Greek yogurt and a dash of honey

Recipes for perimenopause/menopause:

1. Hormone-Balancing Salad:
- Ingredients: Mixed greens, sliced avocado, shredded beetroot, pomegranate seeds, pumpkin seeds, and a drizzle of olive oil and lemon juice.
- Instructions: Combine all ingredients in a bowl, toss gently, and enjoy.

2. Flaxseed Protein Pancakes:
- Ingredients: 2 ripe bananas, 2 eggs, ¼ cup ground flaxseed, ¼ cup whole wheat flour, 1 tsp baking powder, 1 tsp vanilla extract, and a pinch of salt.
- Instructions: Blend all ingredients in a blender until smooth. Cook on a non-stick pan over medium heat, flipping once. Serve with fresh fruits or a dollop of Greek yogurt.

3. Roasted Salmon with Broccoli:
- Ingredients: Salmon fillet, fresh broccoli florets, olive oil, lemon juice, garlic powder, salt, and pepper.
- Instructions: Preheat oven to 400°F (200°C). Place the salmon on a baking sheet, arrange broccoli florets around it. Drizzle olive oil and lemon juice over salmon and broccoli. Season with garlic powder, salt, and pepper. Bake for 15-20 minutes or until salmon is cooked through and broccoli is tender.

Remember, these are just a few ideas to get you started. It's important to consult with a healthcare professional or a registered dietitian to get personalized advice based on your specific needs and preferences.

5.3 Nutritional Considerations for Common Symptoms

Proper nutrition can play a crucial role in managing common symptoms associated with perimenopause and menopause. Here are some key nutritional considerations for specific symptoms:

1. Hot flashes and night sweats: Certain foods may trigger hot flashes, while others can help alleviate them. Avoid spicy foods, caffeine, alcohol, and sugary foods, as they may exacerbate symptoms. Instead, focus on incorporating cooling foods like leafy greens, cucumber, watermelon, and mint. Soy products like tofu and edamame may be beneficial due to their phytoestrogen content.

2. Mood swings and irritability: To support stable moods, include foods rich in B vitamins such as leafy greens, legumes, and whole grains. These nutrients help in the production of neurotransmitters like serotonin, associated with mood regulation. Omega-3 fatty acids found in fatty fish (salmon, sardines) and walnuts may also be beneficial for mood.

3. Joint pain and stiffness: Anti-inflammatory foods can help reduce joint pain and stiffness. Include foods rich in omega-3 fatty acids (fatty fish, chia seeds, flaxseeds), ginger, turmeric, and dark leafy greens. These foods have anti-inflammatory properties and may help alleviate symptoms.

4. Sleep disturbances: Avoid caffeine, especially close to bedtime. Incorporate sleep-promoting foods like cherries, kiwi, jasmine rice, and herbal teas such as chamomile and lavender. Additionally, magnesium-rich foods like dark chocolate, almonds, and leafy greens can support relaxation.

5. Bone health: During menopause, bone density can decrease due to decreasing estrogen levels. Make sure to consume adequate calcium-rich foods like dairy products, sesame seeds, leafy greens, and fortified plant-based milk. Vitamin D plays a crucial role in calcium absorption, so consider getting enough sunlight exposure or incorporating vitamin D-rich foods like fatty fish (salmon, mackerel) and fortified dairy alternatives.

It's important to note that everyone's needs are unique, and it may be beneficial to consult with a registered dietitian who can provide personalized guidance based on your specific symptoms and medical history.

Chapter 7: Self-Care in Perimenopause and Menopause

Self-care is crucial during menopause as it can help manage symptoms, promote well-being, and improve overall quality of life. Here are some self-care practices to consider:

1. Prioritize Rest and Sleep: Menopause can disrupt sleep patterns. Establish a relaxing bedtime routine, create a sleep-friendly environment, and aim for 7-9 hours of quality sleep each night.

2. Engage in Regular Physical Activity: Regular exercise can help manage weight, improve mood, reduce stress, and support bone health. Choose activities you enjoy, such as walking, swimming, yoga, or strength training, and aim for at least 150 minutes of moderate-intensity exercise each week.

3. Manage Stress: Menopause can be a stressful time due to hormonal changes and associated symptoms. Find stress-

management techniques that work for you, such as deep breathing exercises, meditation, mindfulness, or engaging in hobbies and activities that bring you joy.

4. Nurture Relationships: Building and maintaining strong social connections is important for emotional well-being. Seek support from friends, family, or support groups. Sharing experiences and receiving support can make the menopause transition easier.

5. Practice Relaxation Techniques: Incorporate relaxation techniques into your daily routine, such as deep breathing exercises, progressive muscle relaxation, or taking warm baths. These practices can promote relaxation and reduce symptoms like hot flashes and anxiety.

6. Eat a Balanced Diet: Proper nutrition is essential during menopause. Focus on incorporating a variety of whole foods, such as fruits, vegetables, whole grains, lean proteins, and healthy fats. Stay hydrated and limit alcohol, caffeine, and processed foods, as they can exacerbate symptoms.

7. Take Time for Yourself: Engage in activities that bring you joy and relaxation. Whether it's reading, gardening, listening to music, or pursuing creative outlets, carving out time for yourself is essential for self-care.

8. Seek Professional Help: If you're struggling with severe symptoms or finding it difficult to cope, do not hesitate to seek advice from healthcare professionals, such as your primary care physician or a menopause specialist. They can provide guidance and support tailored to your individual needs.

Remember, self-care is a personal journey. It's important to listen to your body, be kind to yourself, and find what practices work best for you.

7.1 The Importance of Self-Care

Self-care is crucial during perimenopause and menopause as these transitional phases can bring about physical and emotional changes. Taking care of yourself can improve your overall well-being and help you navigate through this stage more smoothly. Here are some reasons why self-care is important during perimenopause and menopause:

1. Physical well-being: Menopause is associated with various physical symptoms like hot flashes, night sweats, insomnia, mood swings, and fatigue. Engaging in regular exercise, maintaining a healthy diet, and getting enough sleep can help alleviate these symptoms and improve your physical health.

2. Emotional well-being: Hormonal changes during perimenopause and menopause can lead to mood swings, irritability, anxiety, and depression. Engaging in activities that reduce stress, such as meditation, yoga, or spending time in nature, can help to balance your emotions and support your mental well-being.

3. Hormonal balance: Certain self-care practices can promote hormonal balance during perimenopause and menopause. This includes avoiding excessive caffeine and alcohol, reducing processed foods, and incorporating more fruits, vegetables, and whole grains into your diet. Regular exercise is also beneficial as it helps regulate hormone production.

discuss the potential risks and benefits with your doctor to determine the best course of action for you.

7. Practice good sleep hygiene: Adopting healthy sleep habits is important for quality rest. Avoid caffeine and stimulating activities close to bedtime, limit exposure to electronic screens, and create a before-bed ritual to wind down. Reading a book, practicing light stretching, or listening to soothing music can help signal to your body that it's time to relax and prepare for sleep.

Remember, sleep and rest are crucial for overall health, and during menopause, getting enough rest can help manage the associated symptoms. However, if you continue to experience persistent sleep disturbances or extreme fatigue, it's always a good idea to consult with a healthcare professional for targeted advice and support.

7.3 Cultivating Healthy Habits and Routines

Cultivating healthy habits and routines during perimenopause and menopause can help support physical and mental well-being during this transition. Here are some key points to consider:

1. Regular exercise: Engaging in regular physical activity can help manage weight, improve mood, and relieve menopausal symptoms. Incorporate activities you enjoy, such as walking, swimming, yoga, or strength training, into your routine. Aim for at least 150 minutes of moderate-intensity exercise per week, or as advised by your healthcare provider.

2. Balanced diet: Focus on a nutritious and balanced diet to support hormonal balance and overall health. Include a variety of fruits, vegetables, whole grains, lean proteins, and healthy fats in your meals. Limit processed foods,

sugary snacks, and caffeine, as they can exacerbate menopausal symptoms.

3. Stay hydrated: Hormonal changes during menopause can increase the risk of dehydration. Make sure to drink plenty of water throughout the day to stay properly hydrated. Limit alcohol and caffeine intake, as they can contribute to dehydration and disrupt sleep.

4. Practice stress management: Prioritize stress reduction techniques such as mindfulness, deep breathing exercises, or tai chi. Engaging in activities that help you relax and unwind can be particularly beneficial during this stage. Consider incorporating stress-reducing activities into your daily routine to support emotional well-being.

5. Adequate sleep: As mentioned earlier, prioritize good sleep hygiene and ensure you're getting enough restful sleep. Develop a bedtime routine that promotes relaxation, create a sleep-friendly environment, and maintain a consistent sleep schedule to support optimal sleep quality.

6. Seek emotional support: Menopause can bring about emotional and psychological changes. It's important to seek emotional support from friends, family, or even professionals if needed. Joining support groups or talking to others who are going through similar experiences can provide a sense of community and validation.

7. Regular check-ups: Stay proactive about your health by scheduling regular check-ups with your healthcare provider. Discuss any lingering concerns or menopausal symptoms, and work together to develop a personalized plan to address them. Consider regular screenings, including bone density and breast cancer screenings, as recommended by your healthcare provider.

By cultivating healthy habits and routines, you can support your physical and mental well-being during perimenopause and menopause. Remember, everyone's experience is unique, so it's important to listen to your body and make adjustments as needed. Consulting with a healthcare professional can provide additional guidance and support tailored to your individual needs.

Chapter 8: Nurturing Relationships and Menopause

Of course! Nurturing relationships during perimenopause and menopause is essential for emotional support and overall well-being. Here are some suggestions on how to navigate this stage while maintaining strong relationships:

1. Communication: Open communication is key when dealing with the challenges of perimenopause and menopause. Share your experiences, concerns, and emotions with your loved ones so that they understand what you're going through. This helps them offer support and empathy.

2. Education: Encourage your loved ones to learn about perimenopause and menopause so they have a better understanding of the physical and emotional changes you're experiencing. Provide them with resources or have conversations about the topic to increase their knowledge and sensitivity.

3. Empathy and patience: Understand that perimenopause and menopause can lead to mood swings, irritability, and other changes in behavior. Encourage your loved ones to be patient and empathetic during this time. Remind them that

it's a temporary phase and you would appreciate their understanding.

4. Seeking support together: Attend doctor's appointments or therapist sessions together, if appropriate, to facilitate a deeper understanding of the challenges you're facing. This can help your loved ones actively participate in your healthcare decisions and make them feel included in your journey.

5. Quality time: Prioritize spending quality time with your loved ones. Engage in activities that bring you joy and allow you to connect on a deeper level. This could involve going for walks, doing hobbies together, or simply having heartfelt conversations.

6. Self-care: Remember to take care of yourself during this time. Prioritizing self-care allows you to better nurture your relationships. Engage in activities that help you relax and reduce stress, such as exercising, meditating, or pursuing hobbies you enjoy. When you take care of yourself, you'll be better equipped to maintain healthy relationships.

7. Seek professional help if needed: If you're finding it challenging to manage the emotional and physical changes of perimenopause and menopause, consider seeking professional help. A therapist or counselor experienced in menopause can provide guidance and support for both you and your loved ones.

Remember, nurturing relationships during this stage is about being open, understanding, and patient. By involving your loved ones in your journey and taking care of yourself, you can navigate perimenopause and menopause while strengthening your relationships.

8.1 Communicating with Loved Ones about Menopause

When it comes to discussing perimenopause and menopause with loved ones, open and honest communication is key. Here are some tips and strategies to help you navigate these conversations:

1. Choose the right timing: Find a quiet moment when both you and your loved one are relaxed and have time to talk without distractions. This will create a comfortable environment for sharing and listening.

2. Educate yourself: Before starting the conversation, make sure you understand the topic thoroughly. Research the symptoms, changes, and experiences associated with perimenopause and menopause. This knowledge will help you communicate more effectively.

3. Express your needs: Begin by expressing your own experiences, needs, and concerns. Share the symptoms you're experiencing and how they affect your daily life. Being open and vulnerable can help your loved ones understand what you're going through.

4. Provide information: Sometimes loved ones may struggle to understand what menopause entails. Offer educational resources such as articles, books, or websites that provide accurate and reliable information. This can help them gain a better understanding of the physical and emotional changes you're experiencing.

5. Encourage empathy: Explain how the symptoms of perimenopause or menopause can impact your emotional well-being. Encourage your loved ones to listen and show empathy rather than dismissing or minimizing your

experiences. Helping them see things from your perspective can foster a deeper understanding.

6. Share communication preferences: Let your loved ones know how they can best support you during this time. Share what strategies or approaches work well for you when it comes to having conversations or receiving emotional support. Clear communication can create an environment of understanding and empathy.

7. Invite questions: Open up the dialogue and invite your loved ones to ask questions. Be prepared to answer them honestly and patience, as they may be curious but unsure of how to approach the topic. Encourage an open and non-judgmental atmosphere where they feel comfortable seeking more information.

Remember, everyone's experience with perimenopause and menopause is different, so be patient and understanding in your conversations. By communicating openly and providing accurate information, you can foster a supportive and compassionate environment with your loved ones.

8.2 Navigating Intimacy and Sexuality

Navigating intimacy and sexuality during perimenopause and menopause can bring about various changes and challenges. Here are some suggestions to help you navigate this aspect of your life during this transitional phase:

1. Educate yourself: Become informed about the physical and emotional changes that can occur during perimenopause and menopause. Knowing what to expect can help you feel more confident and better equipped to communicate with your partner.

2. Communication is key: Have open, honest, and non-judgmental conversations with your partner about your experiences. Discuss any concerns, fears, or physical discomfort that you may be experiencing. Sharing your feelings can foster understanding and support between both partners.

3. Explore new approaches: Keep an open mind and consider trying new things in the bedroom. Experiment with different sexual activities, positions, or techniques that may be more comfortable or enjoyable during this phase. Take the time to discover what feels best for you and communicate your preferences to your partner.

4. Prioritize self-care: Practice self-care activities that promote overall well-being, such as regular exercise, stress reduction techniques, and a healthy diet. Taking care of your physical and emotional health can have positive effects on your libido and sexual satisfaction.

5. Seek professional advice: If you're experiencing specific concerns or physical symptoms that are affecting your intimacy, consider seeking guidance from a healthcare professional. They can provide advice, information, and potential solutions to help address any specific challenges you may be facing.

6. Use lubrication: Vaginal dryness is a common symptom during perimenopause and menopause. Using water-based lubricants can help alleviate discomfort during sexual activity. There are various options available over-the-counter, and you can discuss with your healthcare provider for any specific recommendations.

7. Be patient and understanding: Recognize that changes in libido and sexual function are natural during this phase of

life. Be patient with yourself and your partner as you navigate these changes together. It is essential to approach the topic with empathy and kindness, allowing each other space to adjust and explore new ways of connecting intimately.

Remember, every person's experience is unique, so what works for one might not work for another. The key is maintaining open lines of communication with your partner, being willing to explore new approaches, and seeking professional advice when needed. Prioritizing self-care and understanding each other's needs will help you and your partner navigate intimacy and sexuality during perimenopause and menopause.

8.3 Building a Supportive Network

It's important to have a strong support system during this stage of life, as it can bring about various physical and emotional changes. Here are some tips:

1. Open up to friends and family: Share your experiences and struggles with your loved ones. Expressing your feelings and concerns can help them understand what you're going through and provide the support you need.

2. Join support groups: Look for local or online support groups for women going through perimenopause and menopause. These groups offer a safe space to share experiences, exchange advice, and find understanding from those who are facing similar challenges.

3. Seek professional guidance: Consult a healthcare professional, such as a gynecologist or menopause specialist. They can provide valuable information, medical advice, and treatment options to manage symptoms. They

may also be able to recommend support groups or resources that can help you connect with others in similar situations.

4. Connect with online communities: Participate in online forums, social media groups, or specialized websites devoted to perimenopause and menopause. Engaging with these communities can provide a wealth of knowledge, support, and a platform to ask questions from experienced individuals.

5. Educate yourself: Stay informed about the physiological and psychological changes that occur during perimenopause and menopause. Reading books, reputable websites, and articles written by experts can help you better understand the process and make informed decisions.

6. Prioritize self-care: Take time for yourself and engage in activities that promote well-being. This can include physical exercise, meditation, journaling, or pursuing hobbies that bring you joy. Self-care not only improves your overall well-being but also helps reduce stress during this transitional phase.

Remember, building a supportive network is about finding people who can empathize, share knowledge, and offer encouragement. Perimenopause and menopause are natural stages of life, and having support can make the journey smoother and more manageable.

Chapter 9: Alternative Approaches to Menopause

In this chapter, we will explore alternative approaches to perimenopause and menopause, offering a range of options for managing symptoms and promoting overall well-being. Here are some key topics we can cover:

1. Herbal remedies: We'll discuss the use of herbs like black cohosh, dong quai, and red clover, which are known for their potential to alleviate hot flashes, night sweats, and other menopausal symptoms. We'll look at both the scientific evidence supporting their efficacy and any potential risks or side effects associated with their use.

2. Acupuncture: This ancient Chinese practice involves the insertion of thin needles into specific points on the body. We'll explore how acupuncture may help manage menopausal symptoms, such as hot flashes, mood swings, and insomnia. We'll also discuss any scientific evidence supporting its effectiveness and considerations to keep in mind before trying it.

3. Mind-body techniques: Many women find relief from menopausal symptoms through mind-body practices like yoga, meditation, and deep breathing exercises. We'll delve into how these techniques can help alleviate stress, promote hormone balance, and improve overall well-being during perimenopause and menopause.

4. Dietary changes: We'll explore the role of nutrition in managing menopause symptoms. Certain foods, such as soy, flaxseed, and foods rich in phytoestrogens, may offer relief from hot flashes and support hormone regulation. We'll also discuss the importance of maintaining a well-balanced diet during this transition and provide tips on incorporating these foods into your daily meals.

5. Bio-identical hormone therapy: We'll explore the concept of bio-identical hormones and discuss their potential benefits and risks. Bio-identical hormones are

derived from plant sources and are thought to be more similar to the hormones naturally produced by the body. We'll look at the available forms of bio-identical hormone therapy and highlight key considerations when considering this option.

6. Lifestyle adjustments: Beyond alternative therapies, we'll touch on the importance of adopting a healthy lifestyle during perimenopause and menopause. This includes regular exercise, managing stress effectively, getting adequate sleep, and maintaining a supportive social network. These lifestyle adjustments can significantly impact the experience of menopause and promote overall well-being.

9.1 Herbal Remedies and Supplements

Here are some commonly used herbal remedies and supplements:

1. Black cohosh: Black cohosh is widely used to manage menopausal symptoms, especially hot flashes. It is thought to have estrogen-like effects that may help to balance hormone levels. However, while many women find relief with black cohosh, the scientific evidence is mixed, and more research is needed to fully understand its effectiveness and safety.

2. Dong quai: Dong quai has long been used in traditional Chinese medicine to regulate hormones and relieve menopausal symptoms. It is believed to have estrogen-like effects and can possibly help with hot flashes, vaginal dryness, and mood swings. However, caution should be exercised since it may interact with certain medications and its safety during pregnancy has not been established.

3. Red clover: Red clover contains compounds called isoflavones, which act like weak estrogens in the body. Isoflavones may help alleviate menopausal symptoms, particularly hot flashes and night sweats. As with other herbal remedies, the evidence supporting its effectiveness is inconsistent, and some women may experience side effects like nausea or headache.

4. Evening primrose oil: Evening primrose oil is a popular supplement that contains a fatty acid called gamma-linolenic acid (GLA). Some women use it to manage menopausal symptoms such as breast pain, mood swings, and hot flashes. However, the research on its effectiveness is limited, and it may not work for everyone. It's also important to note that evening primrose oil can interact with certain medications, so it's best to consult with a healthcare professional before using it.

5. Phytoestrogenic supplements: Phytoestrogens are plant compounds that have a weak estrogen-like effect in the body. Supplements such as soy isoflavones, flaxseed, and red clover extract are rich in phytoestrogens. They are believed to help balance hormone levels and alleviate menopausal symptoms. However, it's important to remember that phytoestrogens may not be suitable for everyone, especially those with hormone-sensitive conditions or a history of certain cancers. Consulting with a healthcare professional is essential before incorporating these supplements into your routine.

It's important to approach herbal remedies and supplements with caution. Just because a product is natural does not necessarily mean it is safe or effective. Always talk to your healthcare provider before trying any new herbal remedy or supplement, as they can provide personalized advice and help you navigate potential interactions or contraindications based on your specific health needs.

9.2 Acupuncture, Traditional Chinese Medicine, and Ayurveda

Acupuncture, Traditional Chinese Medicine (TCM), and Ayurveda are alternative approaches that some women consider for managing symptoms during perimenopause and menopause. Here's a brief overview of each:

1. Acupuncture: Acupuncture is an ancient Chinese practice that involves inserting thin needles into specific points on the body. It is thought to stimulate energy flow and promote balance within the body. Some women find that acupuncture can help manage menopausal symptoms, such as hot flashes, night sweats, mood swings, insomnia, and vaginal dryness. While research on acupuncture for menopause is still limited, some studies suggest that it may offer relief for certain symptoms. It's important to consult with a qualified acupuncturist who specializes in women's health to discuss your specific symptoms and treatment options.

2. Traditional Chinese Medicine (TCM): TCM is a comprehensive system of healing that includes acupuncture, herbal medicine, dietary therapy, and other practices. In TCM, menopause is seen as a natural transition that can be supported through balancing the body's energy and nourishing the organs. Traditional Chinese herbal formulas are often prescribed to address specific symptoms like hot flashes, sleep disturbances, and mood swings. The individualized approach of TCM takes into account a person's overall health and aims to restore balance. Consult with a licensed TCM practitioner to discuss how this approach may be tailored to your needs.

3. Ayurveda: Ayurveda is a traditional Indian system of medicine that focuses on balancing the body, mind, and spirit. Like TCM, it takes a holistic approach to menopause management. Ayurvedic treatments may include herbal remedies, dietary recommendations, lifestyle adjustments, meditation, and yoga. Ayurvedic herbs like ashwagandha, shatavari, and brahmi may be used to support hormonal balance and overall well-being during perimenopause and menopause. It is important to consult with an Ayurvedic practitioner who can assess your individual constitution (dosha) and recommend appropriate treatments.

While these alternative approaches can offer potential benefits, it's crucial to remember that they may not work for everyone, and evidence supporting their effectiveness can vary. It's important to consult with qualified practitioners and inform your healthcare provider about any complementary therapies you are considering to ensure coordinated and safe care. Integrating these approaches with conventional medical strategies may provide a more comprehensive approach to managing menopause symptoms.

9.3 Exploring Integrative Therapies

Perimenopause and menopause are stages in a woman's life that involve hormonal changes and can bring about various physical and emotional symptoms. Exploring integrative therapies during this time can be beneficial. Here are some integrative approaches that women often consider:

1. Acupuncture: Acupuncture involves the insertion of thin needles into specific points on the body. It may help relieve hot flashes, night sweats, mood changes, and sleep

disturbances associated with perimenopause and menopause.

2. Herbal supplements: Certain herbs, such as black cohosh, red clover, and evening primrose oil, have been traditionally used to alleviate menopausal symptoms. However, it's essential to consult with a healthcare provider before starting any herbal supplements to ensure they won't interfere with other medications or medical conditions.

3. Mind-body techniques: Practices like meditation, yoga, tai chi, and deep breathing exercises can help manage stress, improve sleep quality, and promote overall well-being during perimenopause and menopause. These techniques have been found to have positive effects on mood, hot flashes, and quality of life.

4. Lifestyle modifications: Making healthy lifestyle choices can greatly impact how women experience perimenopause and menopause. Regular exercise, a balanced diet rich in fruits and vegetables, adequate hydration, and sufficient sleep can contribute to overall well-being.

5. Cognitive-behavioral therapy (CBT): CBT is a form of talk therapy used to treat various conditions, including menopausal symptoms. It focuses on identifying and changing negative thought patterns, improving coping strategies, and managing emotions.

Remember, it's essential to consult with your healthcare provider before starting any new therapies or supplements, as they can provide personalized advice based on your medical history and individual needs. Integrative therapies can be helpful in managing perimenopausal and menopausal symptoms, but individual experiences may vary.

Chapter 10: Embracing Your Perimenopause and Menopause Journey

Embracing change and practicing self-acceptance during perimenopause and menopause can be transformative experiences. Here are a few key points to consider:

1. Embracing Change: Menopause is a natural and inevitable phase of a woman's life. It brings about a variety of changes, both physical and emotional. Embracing these changes is essential for maintaining a positive mindset. Rather than resisting or viewing menopause as a negative event, try to reframe it as a new chapter full of opportunities for personal growth and self-discovery.

2. Self-Acceptance: Menopause can sometimes be accompanied by feelings of loss or a sense of not being in control of your body. However, practicing self-acceptance is crucial during this time. Focus on embracing your body and its natural processes. Celebrate the wisdom and experience that comes with age, and recognize that menopause is a normal part of the journey towards self-fulfillment.

3. Education and Awareness: Educating yourself about the physical and emotional changes that occur during perimenopause and menopause can help you better understand what you're experiencing. Stay informed about the various symptoms, such as hot flashes, mood swings, and changes in libido. By becoming more aware, you can adapt your lifestyle and seek necessary support or treatments when needed.

4. Self-Care and Lifestyle Modifications: During menopause, taking care of yourself becomes increasingly important. Prioritize self-care activities that promote overall well-being, such as regular exercise, balanced nutrition, and stress management techniques like meditation or yoga. Avoiding triggers like caffeine and alcohol could also help minimize some symptoms. Remember, self-care is not selfish; it is an essential aspect of maintaining your physical and mental health during this transitional period.

5. Seek Support: Reach out to friends, family, or support groups who are going through similar experiences. Connecting with others can provide a sense of belonging and make you feel less alone. Consider discussing your experiences with your healthcare provider, who can offer guidance, support, and potentially recommend appropriate treatments to manage any challenging symptoms.

Remember that every woman's experience with perimenopause and menopause is unique. Embracing change and practicing self-acceptance are ongoing processes, so be patient and kind to yourself along the way.

9.1 Embracing Perimenopause and Menopause as a Time of Personal Growth

Embracing perimenopause and menopause as a time of personal growth can be a transformative and empowering experience. Here are a few key points to consider:

1. Embracing Transition: Perimenopause and menopause mark a significant transition in a woman's life. Instead of resisting or viewing it as a negative phase, consider reframing it as an opportunity for personal growth. Embrace the changes your body is going through and

approach them with curiosity and openness. Recognize that you have the power to shape your experience and create positive changes in your life.

2. Self-Reflection and Self-Discovery: Menopause often coincides with a time of self-reflection and reevaluation of priorities. Use this phase as an invitation to explore your desires, goals, and aspirations. Assess your values, strengths, and passions, and consider how you can integrate them into this new chapter of your life. Menopause can provide the space for self-discovery and the chance to align your life with your authentic self.

3. Reinventing Your Identity: Menopause can be an excellent opportunity to redefine your identity. Let go of societal expectations and embrace the freedom to be your true self. Explore new interests, engage in creative endeavors, and pursue activities that bring you joy and fulfillment. Use this phase to tap into your inner wisdom and become the person you've always aspired to be.

4. Embracing Emotional Growth: Menopause can bring about a range of emotions, from joy and confidence to anxiety and sadness. Embrace these emotional experiences as opportunities for growth and self-understanding. Explore healthy coping mechanisms such as therapy, journaling, or practicing mindfulness to navigate any challenging emotions. This emotional growth can deepen your self-awareness and resilience.

5. Prioritizing Self-Care: Use this phase as an opportunity to prioritize self-care and nurture your physical, emotional, and mental well-being. Engage in activities that promote relaxation, such as meditation, yoga, or spending time in nature. Prioritize sleep, maintain a balanced diet, and

engage in regular exercise. Taking care of yourself allows you to show up fully in every aspect of your life.

6. Seeking Knowledge and Connections: Educate yourself about perimenopause and menopause to better understand what to expect. Knowledge helps dispel myths and empowers you to make informed decisions about your health and well-being. Seek out connections with like-minded individuals who can provide support and share insights from their own experiences. Engaging in open conversations can provide a sense of community and support.

9.2 Resources and Support for Your Perimenopause and Menopause Journey

Finding resources and support during your perimenopause and menopause journey is crucial. Here are some valuable options to consider:

1. Healthcare Providers: Consult with your healthcare provider, specifically a gynecologist or menopause specialist, who can provide expertise and guidance. They can help address your concerns, recommend appropriate treatments or therapies, and monitor your overall health during this transition. Regular check-ups and open communication are essential. There is no shame to look for a provider who will listen and validate your symptoms. Not all providers are up to speed with latest science, it might take some time to find one that will listen.

2. Online Communities and Support Groups: Joining online communities or support groups dedicated to menopause can connect you with others who are going through similar experiences. Platforms like Facebook groups, forums, or dedicated websites can provide a safe

space to share stories, seek advice, and find emotional support.

3. Menopause Organizations and Websites: Look for reputable menopause organizations and websites that offer comprehensive information and resources. Examples include the North American Menopause Society (NAMS), International Menopause Society (IMS), or local menopause support groups in your area. These organizations often provide educational materials, expert advice, and access to support networks.

4. Books and Podcasts: Numerous books and podcasts offer valuable insights and guidance on perimenopause and menopause. They cover a wide range of topics, from understanding symptoms to self-care practices and lifestyle modifications. Some popular titles include "The Wisdom of Menopause" by Dr. Christiane Northrup and "The Menopause Manifesto" by Dr. Jen Gunter.

5. Therapy and Counseling Services: Consider engaging in therapy or counseling to navigate the emotional and psychological aspects of perimenopause and menopause. Talking to a professional can help you develop coping strategies, manage stress, and address any underlying emotional challenges that may arise during this phase.

6. Lifestyle and Wellness Apps: Explore available apps focused on menopause management, such as symptom trackers, meditation guides, or exercise programs. These apps can help you monitor your symptoms, implement self-care practices, and provide valuable insights into your overall well-being.

7. Local Support Groups: Research if there are local menopause support groups or women's health

organizations in your community. These in-person groups can offer a safe and supportive environment for sharing experiences, accessing resources, and building connections with others who understand what you're going through.

Remember, finding the right resources and support may take some exploration and trial and error. Don't hesitate to seek out multiple avenues until you find the resources that resonate with you and meet your specific needs. Engaging with a supportive community can make your menopause journey feel less isolating and provide you with the tools and knowledge to navigate this phase with confidence.

Conclusion

"Vibrant Transitions: Unleashing Your Vitality through Perimenopause and Menopause" is an empowering and invaluable resource for women navigating the transformative journey of perimenopause and menopause. Offering a wealth of knowledge, this book sheds light on the physical and emotional changes that occur during this phase of life and provides practical strategies for reclaiming vitality.

The author delves into the importance of fitness, nutrition, and hormone balance, recognizing their pivotal role in supporting women's overall well-being. By emphasizing the connection between these factors and their impact on a woman's vitality, the book provides actionable steps that readers can implement in their daily lives.

Supported by the latest scientific research, the book guides readers through various exercises, dietary recommendations, and lifestyle adjustments tailored specifically to address perimenopause and menopause. By arming women with knowledge and understanding, it empowers them to take control of their health and make informed decisions, ultimately enhancing their overall quality of life during this critical life stage.

Throughout the book, the author adopts a compassionate and supportive tone, acknowledging the unique experiences each woman may face during perimenopause and menopause. By addressing common concerns and providing educated advice, "Vibrant Transitions" serves as a reassuring companion, instilling confidence and self-awareness.

Ultimately, "Vibrant Transitions: Unleashing Your Vitality through Perimenopause and Menopause" is a comprehensive and insightful guide that equips women with the tools to navigate the challenges of perimenopause and menopause. It inspires individuals to reclaim their vitality, embrace their bodies, and thrive during this transformative phase of life.